Newman's

Certified EKG Technician

Study Guide

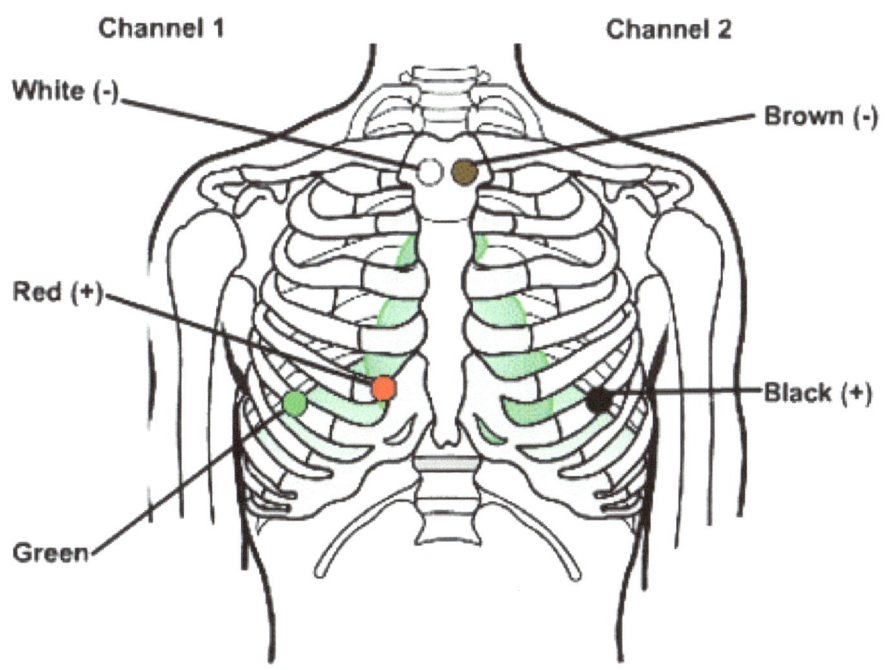

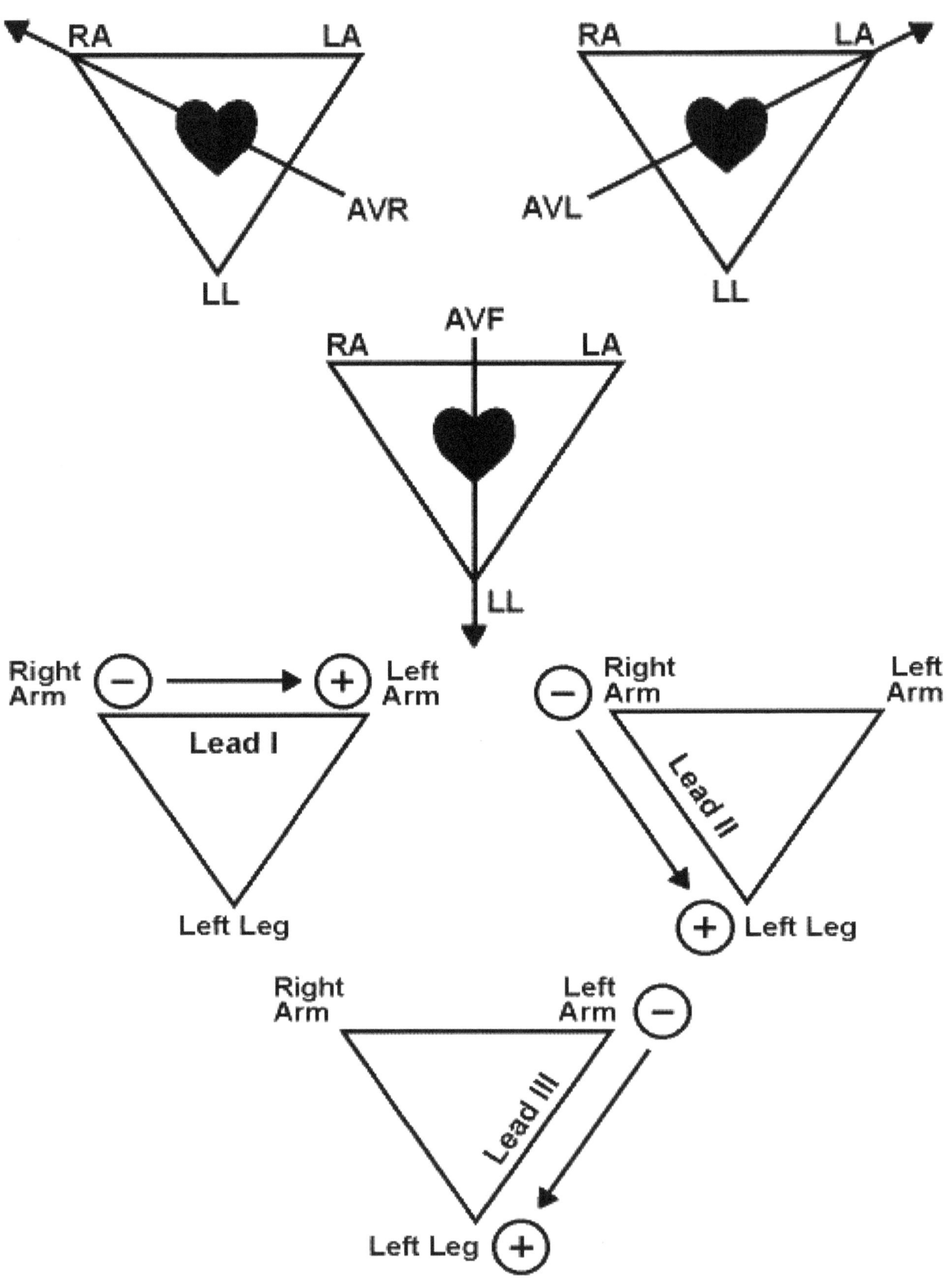

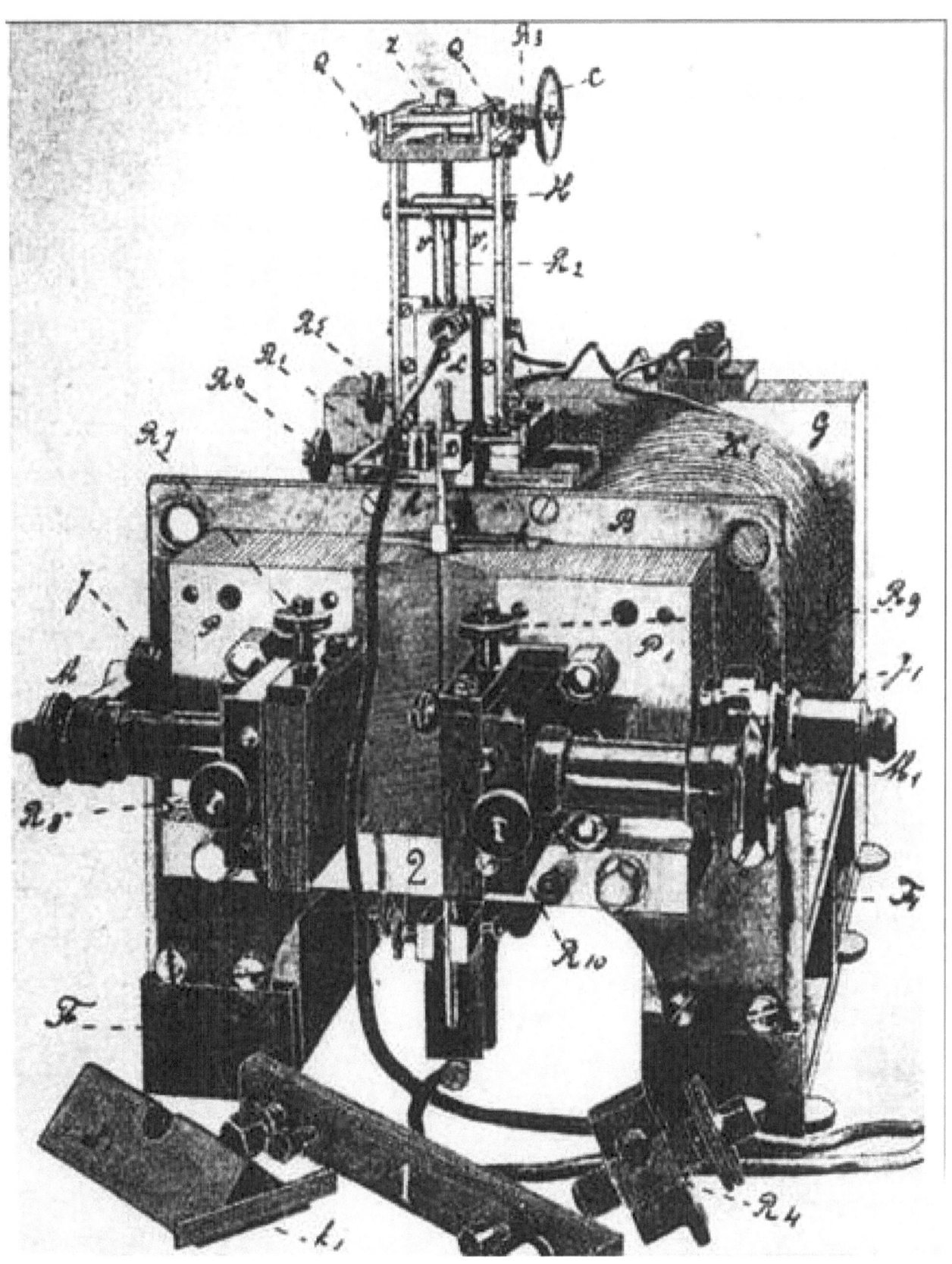

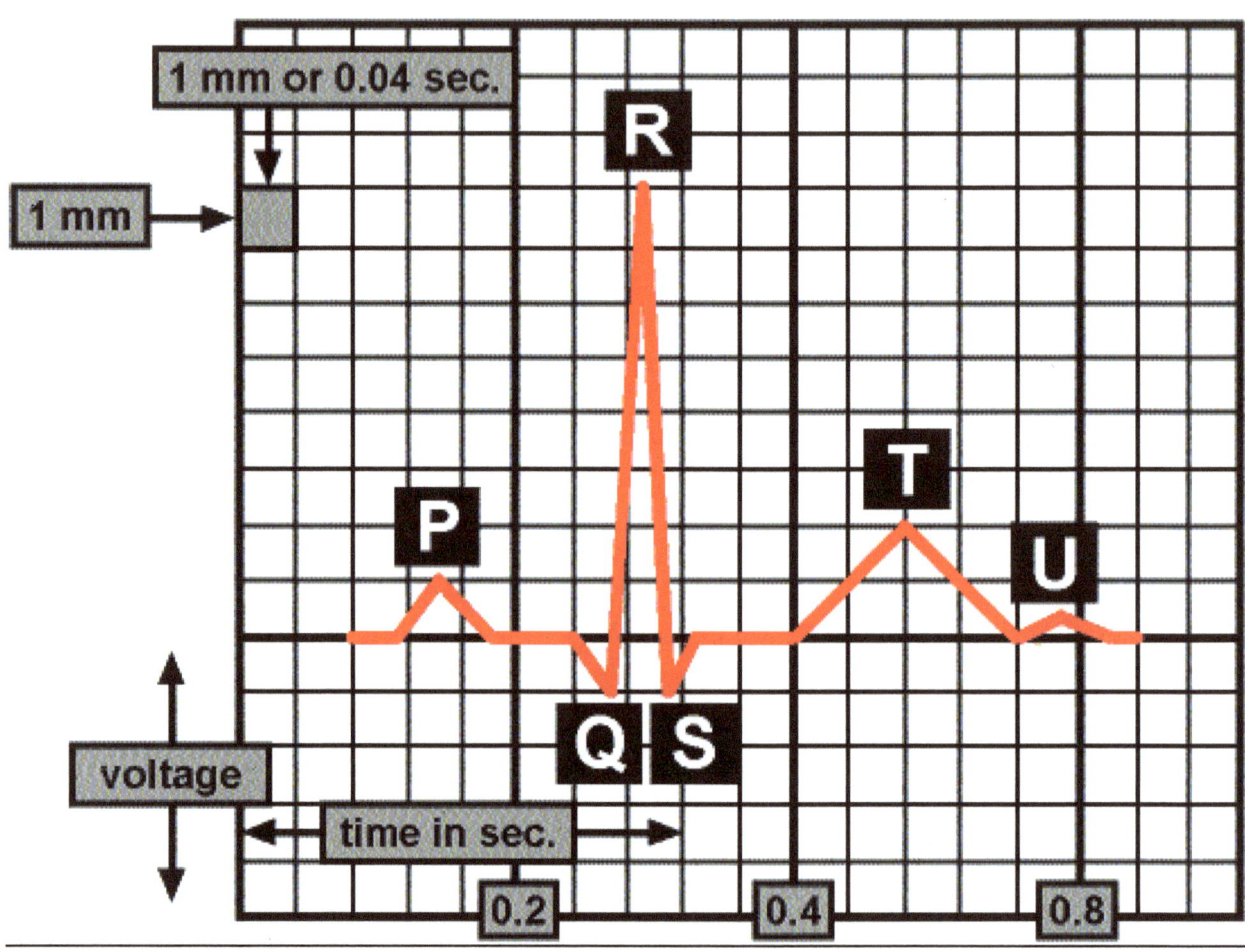

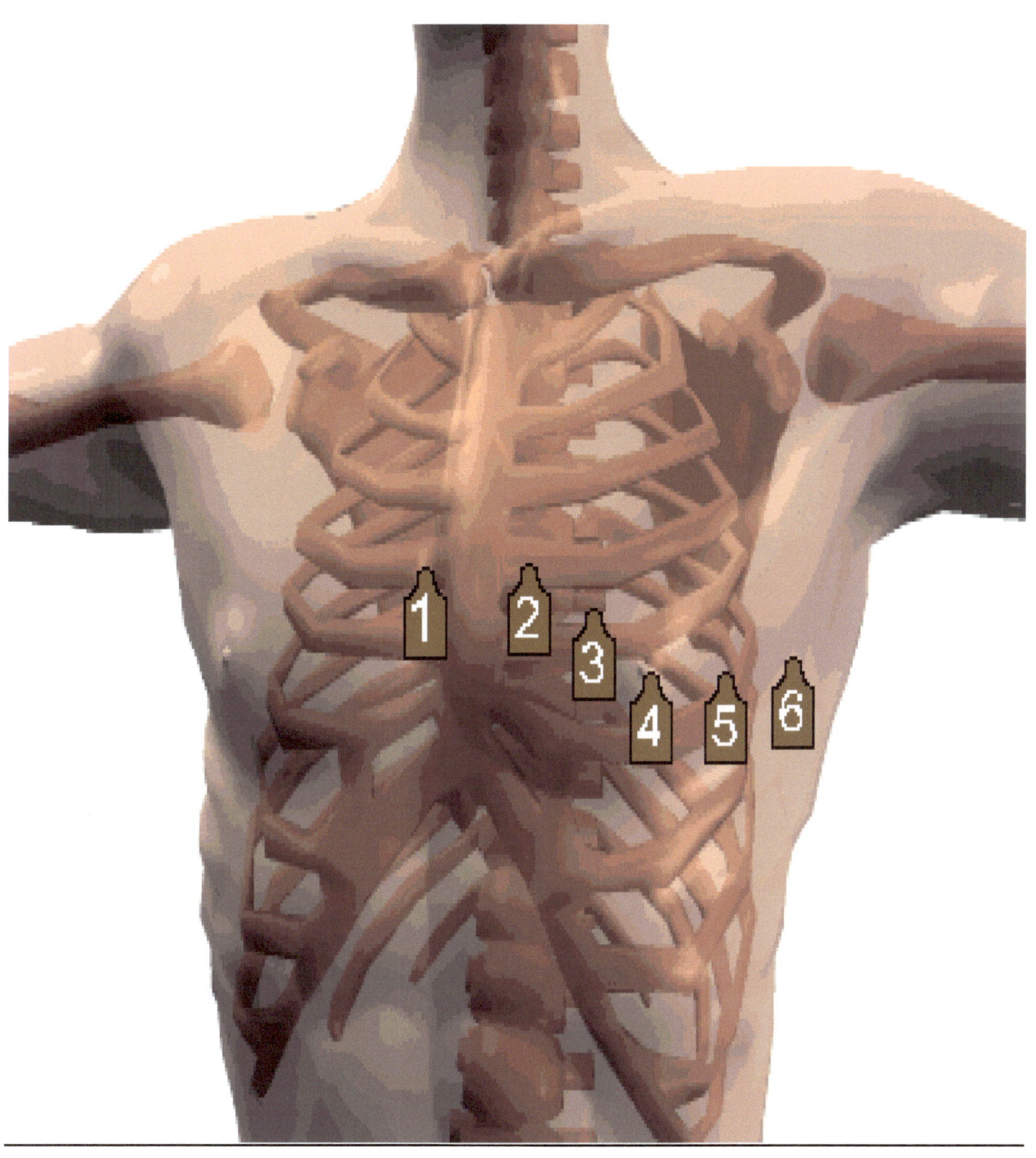

Table of contents

Anatomy of the heart 7
Figure 1: Human Heart 9
Basic Electrophysiology 9
Conduction System of the Heart 10
Figure 2: Conduction System of the Heart 11
Fundamentals of electrocardiogram 11
Figure 3: Precordial Leads 12
The electrocardiographic grid 13
Figure 4: EKG Grid 13
Waves, segments and intervals 13
The Normal Electrocardiogram Complexes 14
Artifacts 15
Stress Testing 15
Exercise stress test 16
Pharmacologic stress test 16
Arrhythmias 16
Myocardial Ischemia and Infarction 16
Ambulatory EKG Monitoring 17
Artifacts of ambulatory EKG recording 18
Event Monitoring 18
Common Cardiovascular Agents 26
Infection Control/Chain Of Infection 28
Legal Considerations 31
Resources: 31
Reference books: 31
Sample EKG Exam 32
Answer Key: 34

Anatomy of the heart
The heart is a hollow muscular organ located in the thoracic cavity between the lungs just behind the sternum.

Layers of the heart
- Endocardium - the innermost layer of the heart. It forms the lining and folds back onto itself to form the four valves. It is in this layer that the conduction system is found.
- Myocardium - the middle and contractile layer of the heart. It is made up of striated muscle fibers interspersed with intercalated disks.
- Epicardium – the outermost layer of the heart. It is actually the inner (visceral) layer of the pericardium.

The Pericardium
The pericardium is a sac in which the heart is contained. It consists of the outermost fibrous pericardium and the serous pericardium which consists of a visceral and a parietal portion. The visceral layer invests the heart and is also called the epicardium. The parietal layer lines the fibrous pericardium. Between the visceral and parietal layers is a serous fluid which serves to prevent friction as the heart beats.

The Heart Chambers
- *Right Atrium* – receives deoxygenated blood returning to the heart from the body via the superior vena cava which carries blood from the upper body and the inferior vena cava which carries blood from the lower body.
- *Right ventricle* – receives deoxygenated blood from the right atrium which it pumps to the lungs for oxygenation through the pulmonary artery (trunk) to the right and left pulmonary arteries.
- The *pulmonary arteries* are the only arteries in the body the carry deoxygenated blood.
- *Left atrium* – receives oxygenated blood returning from the lungs via the right and left pulmonary veins.
- The *pulmonary veins* are the only veins in the body that carry oxygenated blood.
- *Left ventricle* – receives the oxygenated blood from the left atrium and pumps it to the body through the aorta, the largest artery of the body.
- The heart is actually a two-sided pump separated by a septum. The upper chambers consist of the right and left atria (singular: atrium); the lower chambers are the right and left ventricles. The chambers pump simultaneously – both atria contract together then the two ventricles.

Beginning with the right atrium, trace the normal pathway of blood flow through the heart and pulmonary circulation.

_____ Right atrium
_____ Mitral valve
_____ Aorta
_____ Right ventricle
_____ Pulmonic valve
_____ Left atrium
_____ inferior vena cava
_____ Pulmonary trunk
_____ lungs
_____ Left ventricle
_____ Pulmonary arteries
_____ Tricuspid valve
_____ Pulmonary veins
_____ Aortic valve
_____ Systemic circulation
_____ superior vena cava
_____ coronary sinus
_____ aortic arch

The Heart Valves:

The purpose of the heart valves is to prevent backflow of blood thereby assuring uni-directional flow thru the heart.

The *atrioventricular* valves (AV): so-called because they are located between the atria and ventricles.
- a.) Tricuspid valve – located between the right atrium and the right ventricle. As the name connotes, it has three cusps.
- b.) Mitral valve – located between the left atrium and the left ventricle. It has two cusps and it also called the bicuspid valve.

The *semilunar* valves: called semilunar because they have half-moon shaped cusps
- a.) Pulmonic valve – located between the right ventricle and the pulmonary trunk.
- b.) Aortic valve - located between the left ventricle and aorta

Murmurs are caused by diseases of the valves or other structural abnormalities.

The heart sounds are produced by the closure of the valves:
        S1 – first heart sound is due to the closure of the mitral and tricuspid valves.
        S2 – second heart sound is due to the closure of the aortic and pulmonic valves.

Vessels of the Heart

The arteries supplying the heart are the right and left coronary from the aorta. The veins accompany the arteries, and terminate in the right atrium.

Neural Influences of the Heart

The heart is influenced by the autonomic nervous system (ANS) which is subdivided into the sympathetic and parasympathetic nervous systems.

Sympathetic nervous system: affects both the atria and the ventricles by increasing heart rate, conduction and irritability.

Parasympathetic nervous system: affects the atria only by decreasing heart rate, conduction and irritability.

Figure 1: Human Heart

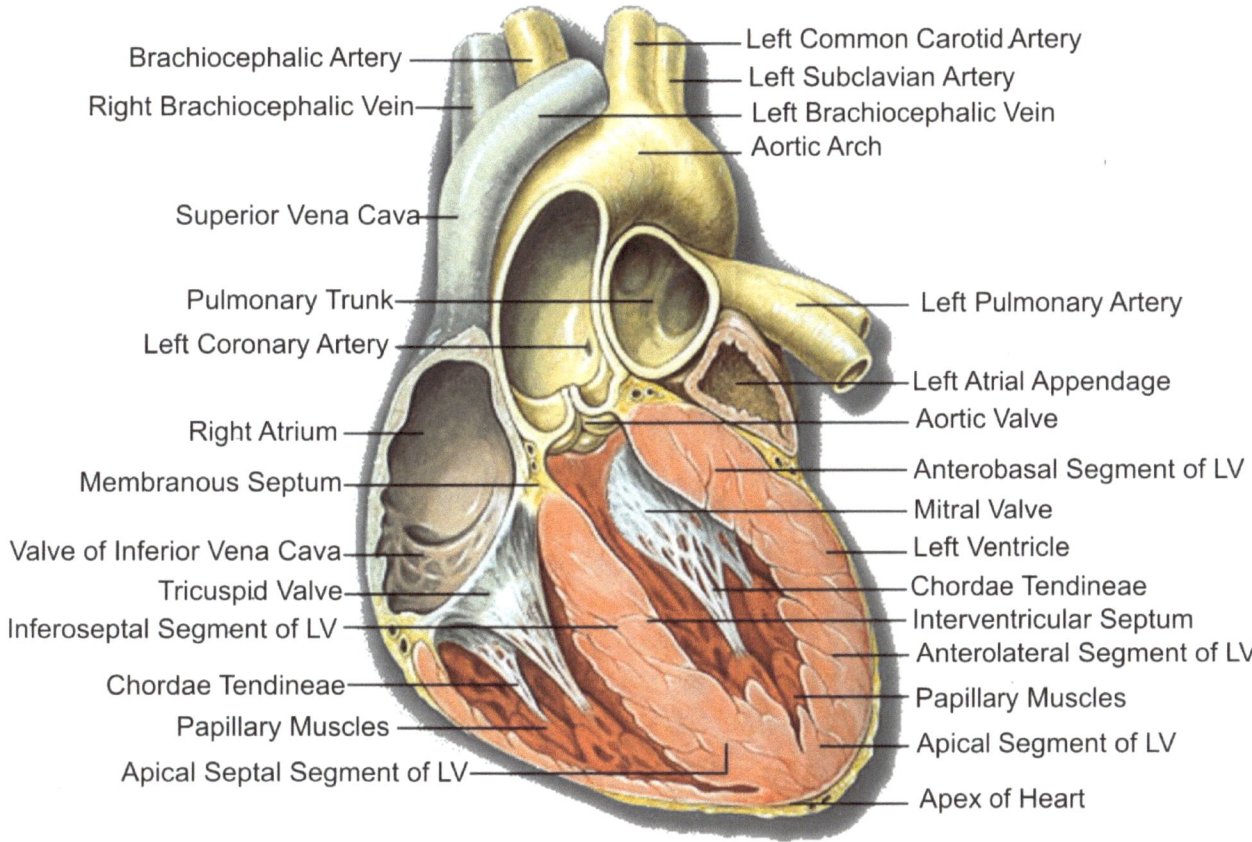

Basic Electrophysiology

Properties of cardiac cells

The primary characteristics of the cardiac cells are:
1. Automaticity – This is the ability of the cardiac pacemaker cells to spontaneously initiate their own electrical impulse without being stimulated from another source. Sites that possess this characteristic are the SA node, AV junction, and the Purkinje fibers.

2. Excitability – Also referred to as irritability. This characteristic is shared by all cardiac cells and it is the ability to respond to external stimulus: electrical, chemical, and mechanical.

3. Conductivity – This is the ability of all cardiac cells to receive an electrical stimulus and transmit the stimulus to the other cardiac cells.

4. Contractility -- This is the ability of the cardiac cells to shorten and cause cardiac muscle contraction in response to an electrical stimulus. This characteristic can be enhanced through administration of certain medications, such as digitalis, dopamine and epinephrine.

Depolarization and Repolarization

Resting cardiac cells are negatively charged inside as compared to the outside. When a cardiac cell is stimulated, sodium ions rush into the cell and potassium leaks out, changing into positive the charge within. This electrical event is called depolarization and is expected to result in contraction. Depolarization flows from the endocardium to the myocardium to the epicardium.

During cell recovery, ions shift back to their original places and the cell recovers the negative charge inside. This is repolarization, and proceeds from the epicardium towards the endocardium. It results in myocardial relaxation.

Conduction System of the Heart

SA Node

Found in the upper posterior portion of the right atrial wall just below the opening of the superior vena cava. It is the primary pacemaker of the heart and has a normal firing rate of 60-100 beats per minute.

Internodal pathways

Consists of anterior, middle and posterior divisions that distribute electrical impulse generated by the SA node throughout the right and left atria to the atrioventricular (AV) node.

AV Junction:
AV node

Located at the posterior septal wall of the right atrium just above the tricuspid valve. There is a $1/10^{th}$ of a second delay of electrical activity at this level to allow blood to flow from the atria to the ventricles.

Bundle of His

Found at the superior portion of the interventricular septum, it is the pathway that leads out of the SA node. It has an ability to initiate electrical impulses with an intrinsic firing rate of 40-60 beats per minute.

Bundle branches

Located at the interventricular septum, the bundle of His divides into the right and left bundle branches, the function of which is to conduct the electrical impulse to the Purkinje fibers.

Purkinje fibers

Found within the ventricular endocardium, it consists of a network of small conduction fibers that delivers the electrical impulses to the ventricular myocardium. This network has the ability to initiate electrical impulses and act as a pacemaker if the higher level pacemakers fail. The intrinsic firing rate is 20-40 beats per minute.

Figure 2: Conduction System of the Heart

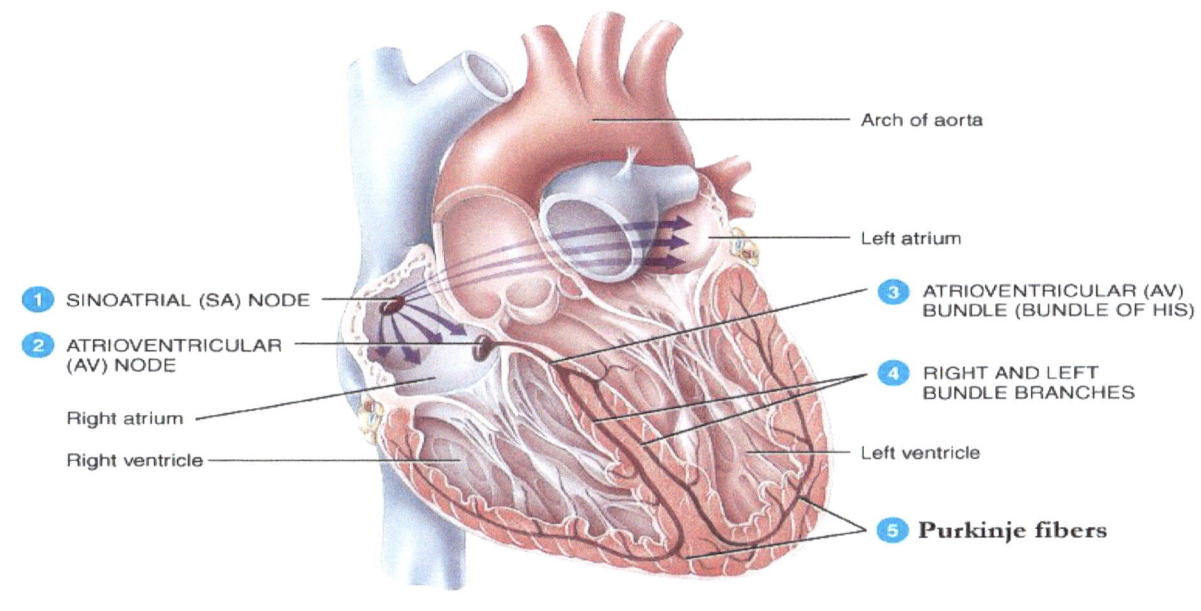

Anterior view of frontal section

Fundamentals of electrocardiogram

Limb Leads:

Consist of three bipolar leads and three augmented leads. These leads record electrical potentials in the frontal plane.

Electrodes are usually applied just above the wrists or upper arms and ankles although the electrical potential recorded will be the same no matter where electrode is placed in the extremity

Bipolar Standard Leads

Electrodes are applied to the left arm (LA), the right arm (RA) and the left leg (LL). Leads are then applied to their respective electrodes. Electrode and lead are also applied to the right leg which acts as a ground (or reference lead) and has no role in production of the electrocardiogram.

        Lead I   = the left arm is positive and the right arm is negative.
                  (LA – RA)
        Lead II = the left leg is positive and the right arm is negative.
                  (LL – RA)
        Lead III = the left leg is positive and the left arm is negative.
                  (LL – LA)

Augmented Unipolar Lead

They are designated as aVR, aVL, and aVF. These leads are unipolar and they require only one electrode from one limb to make a lead. The EKG machine uses a midpoint between the two other limbs as a negative reference point.

Lead aVR = the right arm is positive and the other limbs are negative.
Lead aVL = the left arm is positive and the other limbs are negative.
Lead aVF = the left leg (or foot) is positive and the other limbs are negative.

Unipolar Precordial Leads

Six positive electrodes are placed on the chest to create Leads V1 through V6. They are as follows:

V1 : Fourth intercostal space, right sternal border.
V2 : Fourth intercostal space, left sternal border.
V3 : Equidistant between V2 and V4.
V4 : Fifth intercostal space, left midclavicular line
V5 : Fifth intercostal space, anterior axillary line
V6 : Fifth intercostal space, midaxillary line

Marking Codes

Lead I= •	AVR= −	V1= −•	v4= −••••
Lead II= • •	AVL= − −	V2= −••	v5= −•••••
Lead III= • • •	AVF= − − −	V3= −•••	v6= −••••••

Figure 3: Precordial Leads

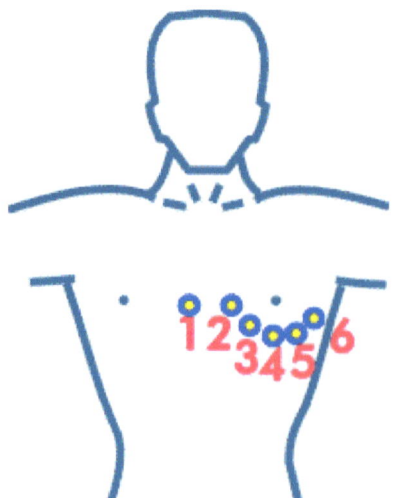

The usual routine EKG consists of placing 10 electrodes on the patient producing 12 Leads: I, II, III, aVR, aVF, aVL; V1-V6.

The electrocardiographic grid

The EKG paper is a graph paper with horizontal and vertical lines at 1-mm intervals. A heavy line appears every 5mm. The horizontal axis represents time: 1mm = 0.04 seconds; 5mm = 0.2 seconds. The vertical axis represents amplitude measured in millivolts but expressed in millimeters: 0.1mV = 1mm. The tracing is marked on the paper by a stylus using heat.

The running speed is 25mm/sec. The EKG machine must be properly standardized so that 1mV will produce a deflection of 10mm.

Figure 4: EKG Grid

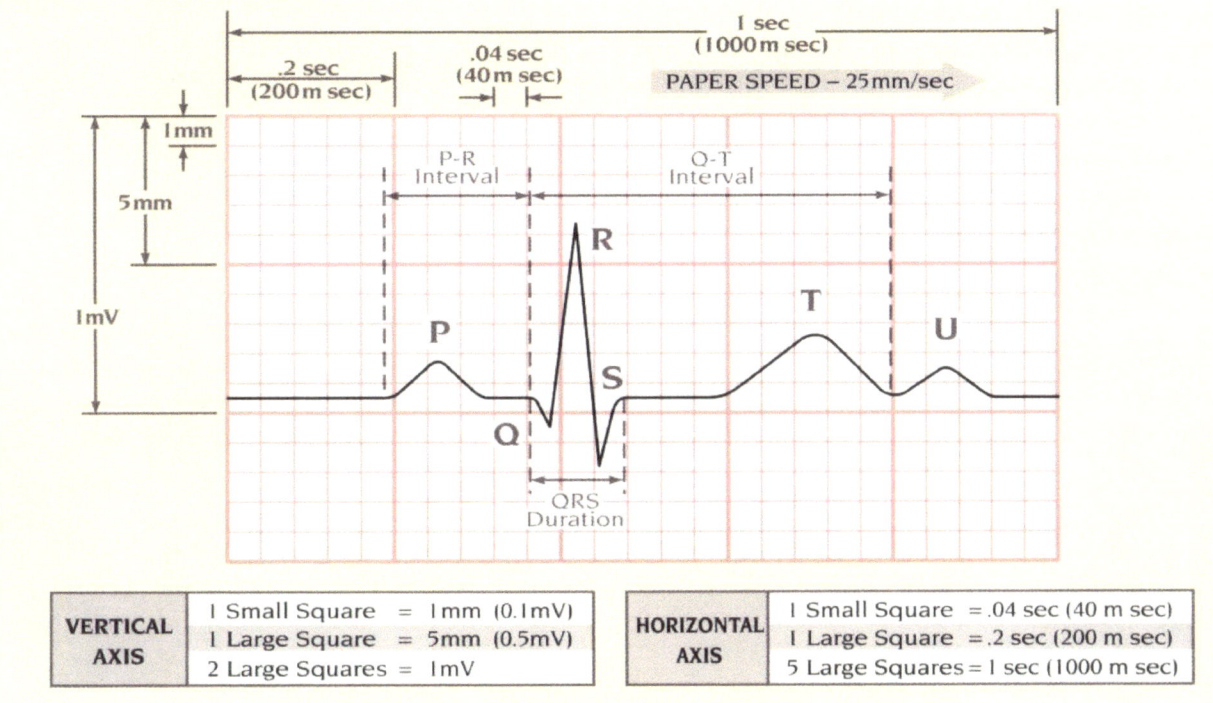

Waves, segments and intervals

- Waveform: refers to movement away from the isoelectric line either upward (positive) deflection or downward (negative) deflection.
- Segment: line between two waveforms.
- Interval: waveform plus a segment.
- Complex: several waveforms

The Normal Electrocardiogram Complexes

Atrial Activation:

P wave: the deflection produced by atrial depolarization. The normal P wave in standard, limb, and precordial leads does not exceed 0.11s in duration or 2.5mm in height.

Ventricular Activation:

- **QRS complex**: represents ventricular depolarization (activation). The ventricle is depolarized from the endocardium to the myocardium, to the epicardium.
- **Q (q) wave**: the initial negative deflection produced by ventricular depolarization.
- **R (r) wave**: the first positive deflection produced by ventricular depolarization.
- **S (s) wave**: the first negative deflection produced by the ventricular depolarization that follows the first positive deflection, (R) wave.

Ventricular Repolarization:

T wave: the deflection produced by ventricular repolarization.
U wave: the deflection seen following the T wave but preceding the next P wave. A prominent is due to hypokalemia (low potassium, blood level).

Normal Intervals:

RR interval: this is the interval between two R waves.

If the ventricular rhythm is regular: the interval in seconds (or fraction of a second) between 2 successive R waves divided into 60 seconds = heart rate/minute. e.g. RR interval of 0.2 sec. (between two heavy lines) = 300/min heart rate; RR interval of 0.8 sec. (between 5 heavy lines) = 75/min heart rate

If the ventricular rhythm is irregular: the number of R waves in six seconds is counted and multiplied by 10 = heart rate/min e.g. 10 R waves occurred within 6 sec. = ventricular rate averages 60/min (10 x 10).

PR interval: P wave plus the PR segment. The normal interval is 0.12 – 0.2 sec.

QRS interval (or duration): represents ventricular depolarization time. It should be no more than 0.1 sec. in the limb leads and 0.11 sec. in the precordial leads.

Normal Segments and Junctions

- PR segment: line from the end of the P wave to the onset of the QRS complex.
- J (RST) junction: point at which QRS complex ends and ST segment begins.
- ST segment: from J point to the onset of the T wave.

Artifacts

Somatic tremors – patient's tremors or shaking the wires can produce jittery patterns on the EKG tracing.

Wandering baseline - sweat or lotion on the patient's skin or tension on the electrode wires can interfere with the signal going to the EKG apparatus causing the baseline of the tracing to move up and down on the EKG paper.

(Alternating current)/60-cycle interference – can produce deflections occurring at a rapid rate that may mimic atrial flutter. This is caused by electrical appliances or an apparatus being used nearby while the tracing is taken.

Broken recording - the stylus goes up and down trying to find the signal. This can be caused by loose electrode or cables or by frayed or broken wires.

Attention to the following will ensure against artifacts and technically poor tracings:

- The patient should be lying on a comfortable bed or table large enough to support the entire body.
- There must be good contact between the skin and the electrode.
- The EKG machine must be properly standardized: 1mV should produce a deflection of 1cm (10mm).
- The patient and the recording machine must be properly grounded to avoid alternating current interference.
- Electronic equipment in contact with the patient can produce artifacts. i.e., IV infusion pumps

Stress Testing

A noninvasive diagnostic procedure to determine the presence and severity of coronary artery disease. The test is performed through exercise (by having the patient walk on a treadmill or by pedaling on a bicycle), or pharmacologically (by administration of medication that causes increase in heart rate), while hooked up to an EKG monitor. The limb leads are applied to the torso of the patient rather than on the extremities themselves. A rhythm strip is run continuously throughout the test and a complete 12-lead EKG is recorded usually every 90 seconds during exercise and every minute in the recovery period post-exercise.

Some indications for stress testing are:
- Evaluation of chest pain in patient with normal EKG.
- Evaluation of patient who has recently had a myocardial infarction.
- Diagnosis and treatment of arrhythmias.

Some indications for terminating the test are:
- Patient develops chest pain, shortness of breath, or dizziness.
- Blood pressure abnormalities

Exercise stress test

This test is performed until at least 85% of the target heart rate is reached or symptoms or EKG changes develop which requires the test to be terminated. Target heart rate is: 220 minus patient's age. For example, the target heart rate for a 40 year old patient is 180 (220 – 40). 85% of 180 or 153 is required for the test to be valid for interpretation.

Pharmacologic stress test

This test is appropriate for patients with physical limitation, e.g. amputees, or those who could not exercise to reach the target heart rate, e.g. elderly. Medications such as adenosine, dipyridamole, or dobutamine are given intravenously through an IV line to cause the heart rate to climb to the target level or the same symptoms and EKG changes as the exercise test develop. The test is concluded after 85% of the target heart rate is achieved.

Arrhythmias

Cardiac arrhythmias are due to the following mechanisms:
1. Arrhythmias of sinus origin - where electrical flow follows the usual conduction pathway but is too fast, too slow, or irregular. Normal sinus rate is 60-100 beats per minute. If the rate goes beyond 100 per minute, it is called sinus tachycardia. If the rate goes below 60 per minute, it is referred to as sinus bradycardia.
2. Ectopic rhythms - electrical impulses originate from somewhere else other than the sinus node.
3. Conduction blocks - electrical impulses go down the usual pathway but encounter blocks and delays.
4. Preexcitation syndromes - the electrical impulses bypass the normal pathway and, instead, go down an accessory shortcut

Myocardial Ischemia and Infarction

Ischemia

Ischemia occurs when there is a decrease in the amount of blood flow to a section of the heart. This is usually experienced as chest pain and discomfort and is called angina.

Myocardial Infarction

Infarction refers to the actual death of the myocardial cells.

The hallmark of infarction on EKG is the presence of abnormal Q waves. Q waves are considered abnormal if they are ≥ 1 mm (0.04 second) wide and the height is greater than 25% of the height of the R wave in that lead. Q waves indicate infarcted or dead myocardial tissue. When the Q waves are combined with changes in T waves and ST segments, they indicate an acute MI.

The World Health Organization (WHO) criteria for the diagnosis of myocardial infarction are the presence of at least two of the following:
- Clinical history of ischemic-type of chest discomfort
- Changes on serial EKG tracings
- Rise and fall in serum cardiac markers

Ambulatory EKG Monitoring

Ambulatory EKG monitoring enables the evaluation of the patient's heart rate, rhythm, and QRST morphology during the usual daily activities.

Holter monitor

This is an ambulatory EKG done to rule out intermittent arrhythmias or ischemia that could be missed on a routine EKG. This may be done as an in-patient or outpatient procedure. The patient is hooked-up to a Holter monitor and EKG signals are recorded on a magnetic tape. After the prescribed duration, the patient returns the monitor to the facility and the tape is entered into a computer and scanned for abnormalities.

Five electrodes are attached to the patient's trunk instead of the arms and leg to prevent muscle artifact. The skin is prepped by abrading a thin layer of skin and then the electrodes are taped to the skin so it will adhere better and prevent from dislodging since the entire procedure will be on for 24 hours or longer. Before the ambulatory recording starts, EKG tracings are taken with the patient lying, sitting, and standing in order to be able to identify these positional changes which can bring about substantial variation in QRST morphology upon playback of the tape.

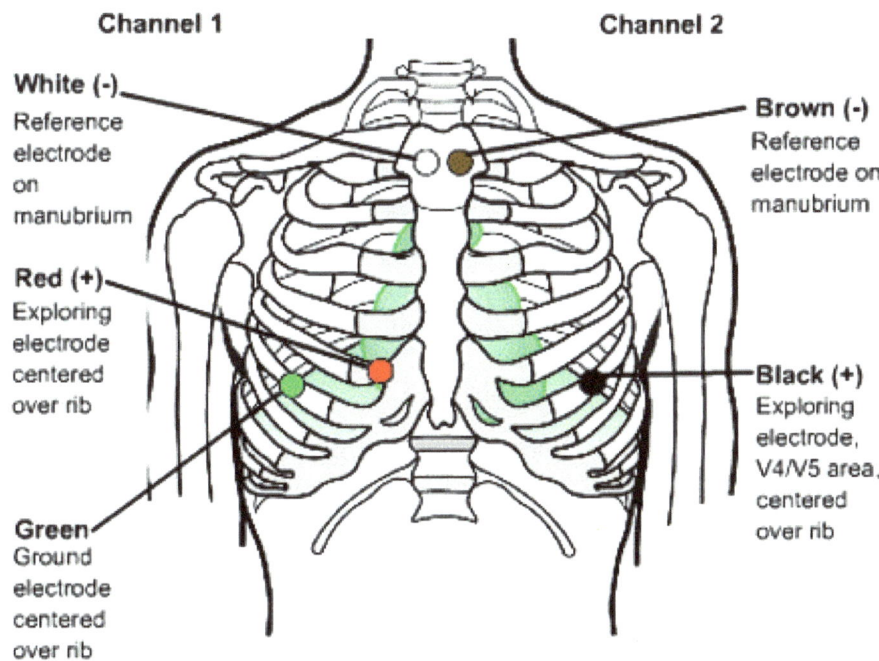

Typical electrode placement for Holter monitoring:

- Two exploring electrodes are placed over bone (to minimize motion artifact) near the V1 (over the 4th or 5th rib to the right of the sternum) and V5 (over the 5th rib at the left midaxillary line).
- Two indifferent electrodes placed over the manubrium
- One ground electrode placed over the 9th or 10th rib at the right midaxillary line

A positive Holter is one that has recorded abnormalities that may explain the patient's symptoms which could include one or more of the following:
- Tachycardias or bradycardias
- ST segment elevation or depression
- Pauses

A negative Holter will have no significant arrhythmias or ST changes.

Artifacts of ambulatory EKG recording
Recording artifacts can result from the following:
- Incomplete tape erasure - this can result in EKG tracings belonging to two different patients confounding both the scanner and the interpreter.
- Tape drag within the apparatus - this will result in recording of spuriously rapid cardiac rhythms. A narrowing of all EKG complexes and intervals should give clue to this situation.
- Battery depletion - this may result in varying QRS amplitude
- Loose connection - intermittently loose connection in the insertion of the electrodes into the recording apparatus can result in the absence of all EKG signals which may mimic bradycardia-tachycardia syndrome. Clue to this artifact is the attenuated QRST morphology of the complexes beginning and ending the pause in rhythm.
- Movement of electrodes - this may occur during scratching the chest near the electrodes and can produce tracings that look like malignant ventricular arrhythmias. However, the underlying rhythm and rate remain undisturbed and should give clue to this artifact.

Event Monitoring
Some patients have symptoms very infrequently that a Holter monitor yields little useful data. These patients are best suited for an event recorder, a hand held device carried in the patient's pocket or purse which is switched only when the patient is actually experiencing the symptom. The EKG is recorded from the anterior chest wall on magnetic tape or computer chip which is scanned later the same way as that of the Holter monitor or it can be transmitted by telephone to a receiving station for immediate attention. Since the event recorder is used only when symptoms occur, multiple recording can be made over the course of a prolonged period of time.

Interpretations

Multiple Choice
Identify the choice that best completes the statement or answers the question.

___ 1. Identify the following rhythm:

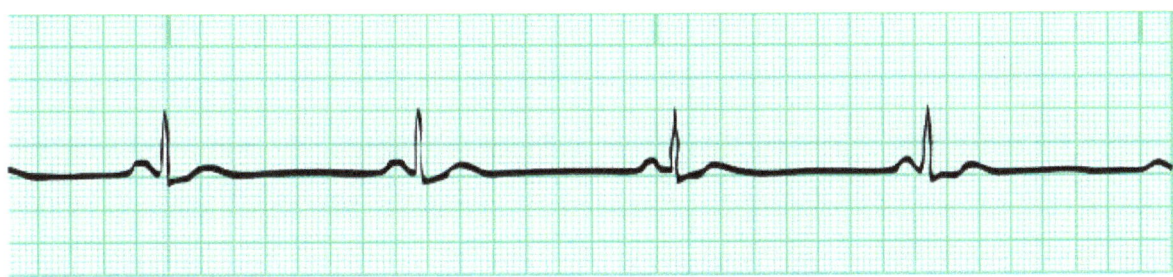

a. sinus bradycardia
b. sinus rhythm
c. sinus tachycardia
d. ventricular bradycardia

___ 2. Identify the following rhythm:

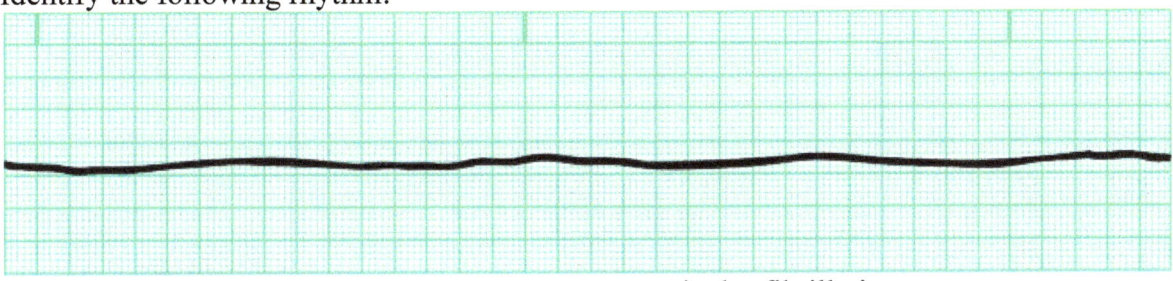

a. ventricular rhythm
b. ventricular tachycardia
c. ventricular fibrillation
d. asystole

___ 3. Identify the following rhythm:

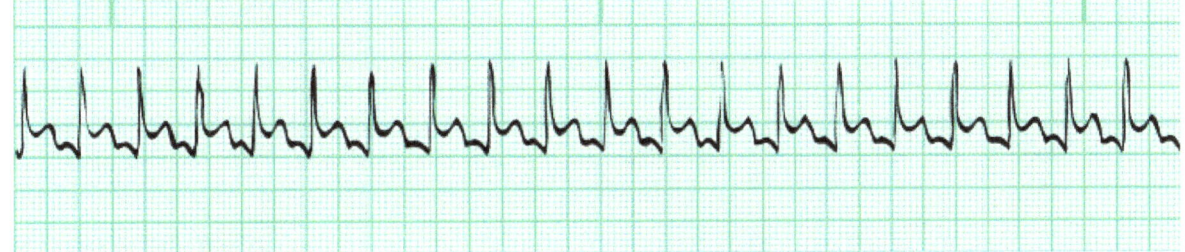

a. atrial fibrillation
b. ventricular tachycardia
c. ventricular fibrillation
d. supraventricular tachycardia (SVT)

___ 4. Identify the following rhythm:

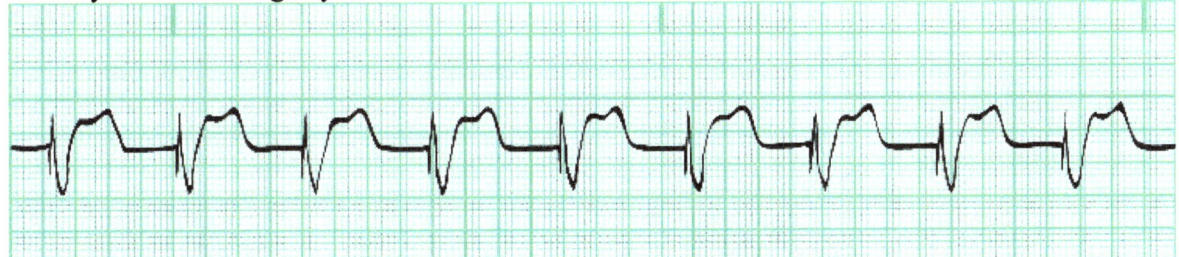

a. atrial fibrillation
b. sinus rhythm
c. bundle branch block
d. pacemaker rhythm

Newman's The Electrocardiographers Study Guide

5. Identify the following rhythm (lead II).

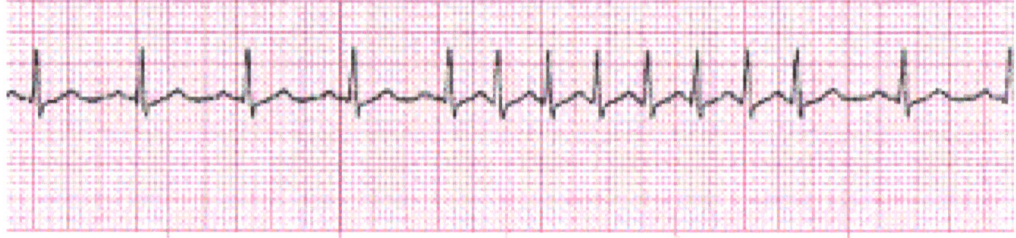

   a. Sinus arrhythmia
   b. Atrial tachycardia
   c. Multifocal atrial tachycardia with a PAC
   d. Sinus rhythm with a PAC, a run of PSVT, back to a sinus rhythm

6. P waves in this rhythm strip:

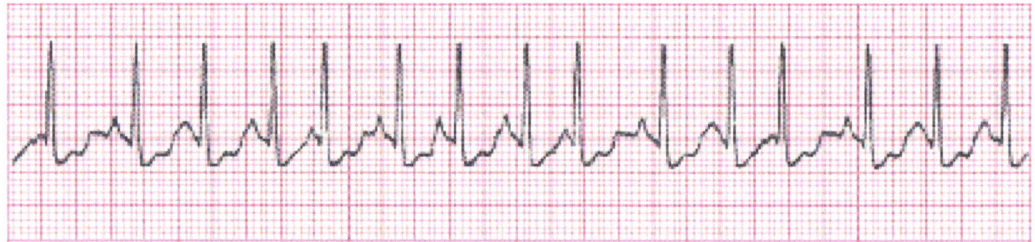

   a. Are upright before every QRS complex.
   b. Are inverted before every QRS complex.
   c. Vary in size and shape.
   d. Are not identifiable.

7. Identify the following rhythm (lead II).

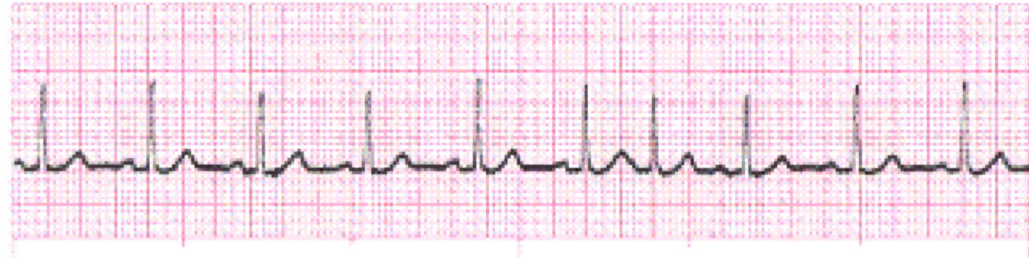

   a. Sinus arrhythmia
   b. Sinus tachycardia
   c. Sinus rhythm with a PAC
   d. Sinus tachycardia with a PAC

8. Identify the following rhythm (lead II).

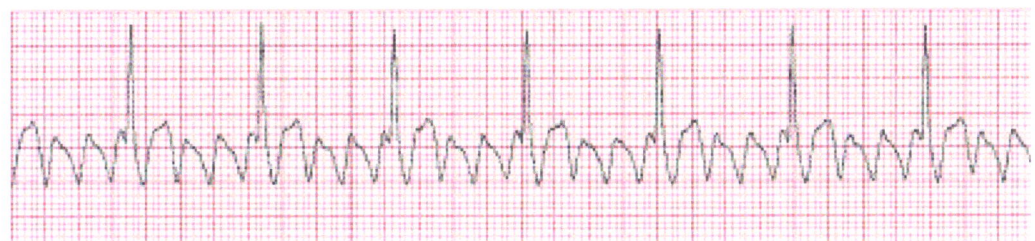

   a. Atrial flutter
   b. Atrial fibrillation
   c. Wolff-Parkinson-White syndrome
   d. AV nodal reentrant tachycardia (AVNRT)

9. Identify the following rhythm (lead II).

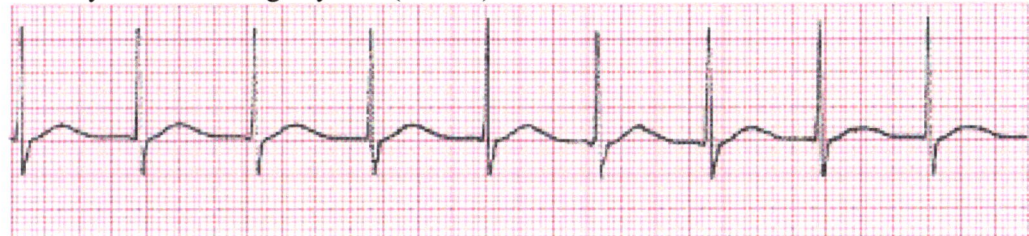

   a. Accelerated junctional rhythm
   b. Sinus rhythm
   c. Junctional rhythm
   d. Sinus arrhythmia

10. Identify the following rhythm (lead II).

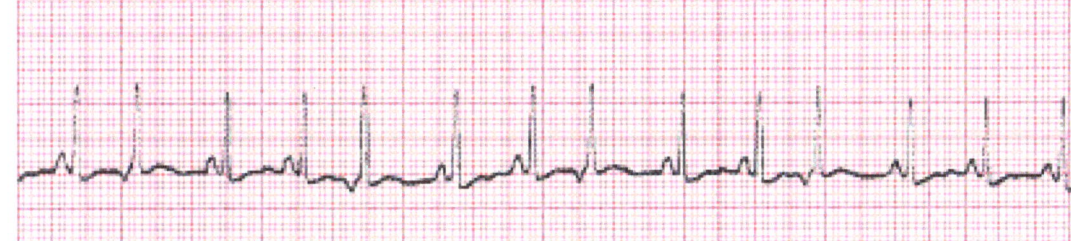

   a. Sinus rhythm with junctional escape beats
   b. Sinus rhythm with PACs
   c. Sinus rhythm with PJCs
   d. Sinus arrhythmia

___ 11. Identify the following rhythm (lead II).

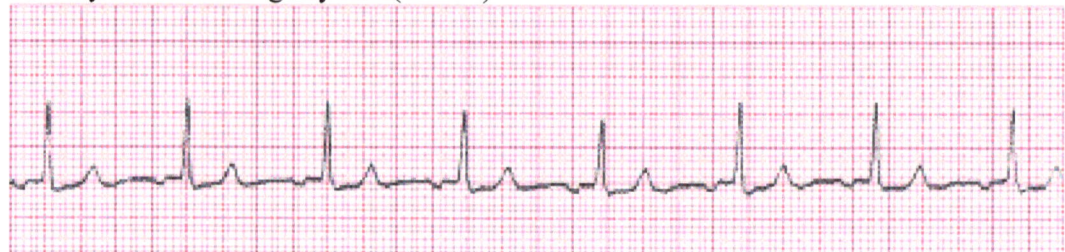

a. Junctional tachycardia
b. Sinus rhythm with PACs
c. Sinus rhythm with PJCs
d. Accelerated junctional rhythm

___ 12. The following rhythm occurred after the patient had recently been treated for a fast heart rate. What should you do now about the patient?

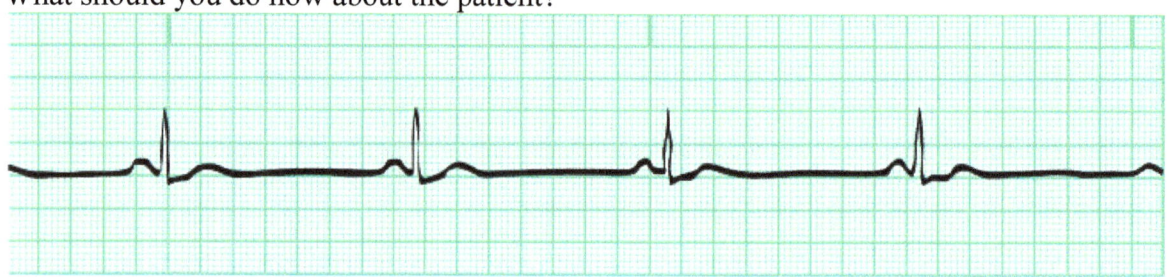

a. no intervention is necessary
b. notify your supervisor immediately
c. check to make sure the patient is not experiencing problems with a low cardiac output.
d. check to make sure that the patient is not experiencing problems with a high cardiac output.

___ 13. Identify the following rhythm:

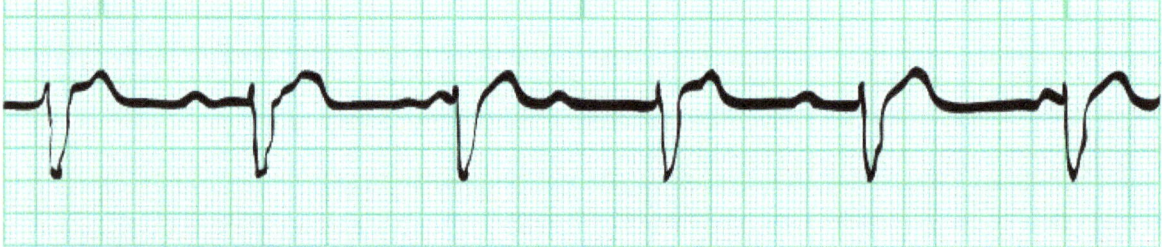

a. Second degree AV block, Mobitz Type I (Wenckeback)
b. Sinus Bradycardia
c. Ventricular rhythm
d. Third Degree AV block - Complete Heart Block

14. Identify the following rhythm:

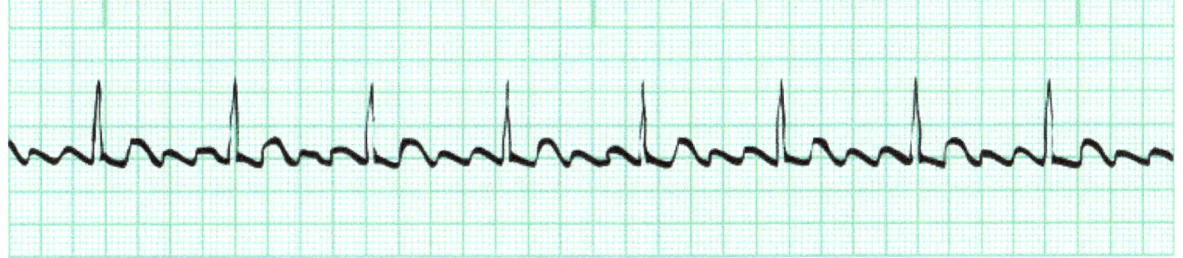

a. Atrial Flutter
b. Atrial Fibrillation
c. Ventricular fibrillation
d. Supraventricular tachycardia (SVT)

28. Identify the following rhythm (lead II):

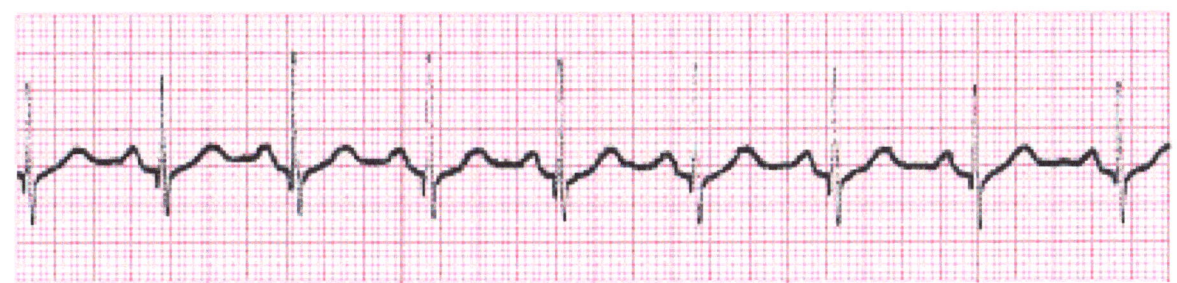

Identification: _____

29. Identify the following rhythm (lead II).

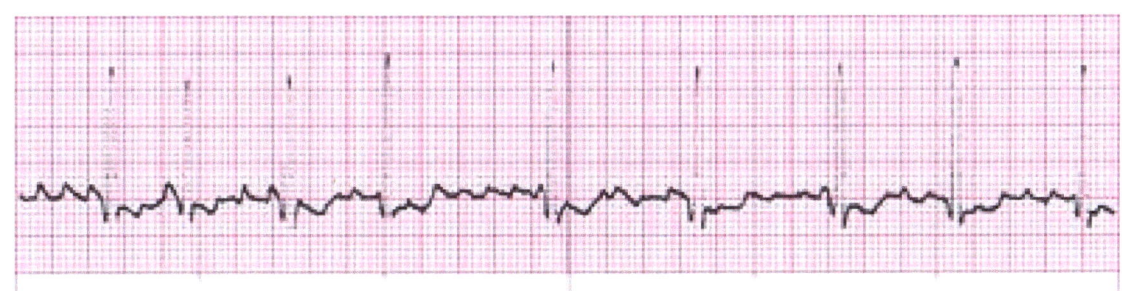

Identification: _____

30. Identify the following rhythm (lead II).

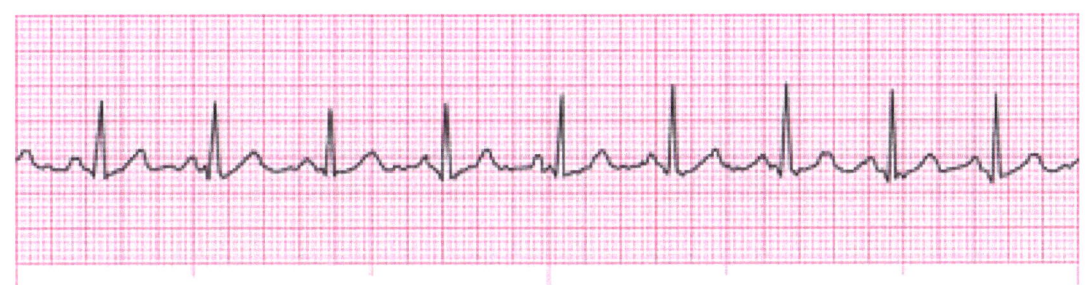

Identification: _____

Newman's The Electrocardiographers Study Guide

31. Identify the following rhythm (lead II).

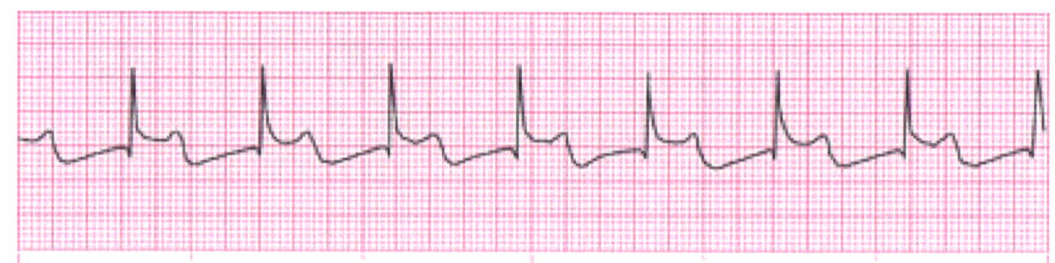

   Identification: _____

34. Identify the following rhythm.

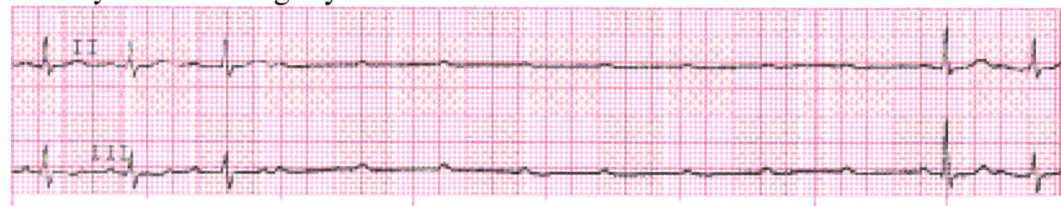

   Identification: _____

35. Identify the following rhythm.

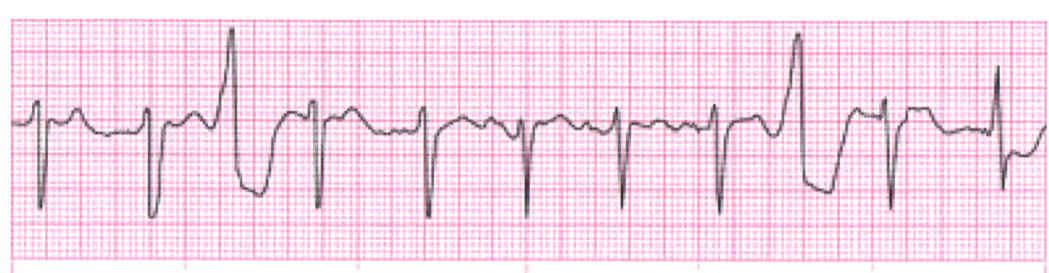

   Identification: _____

36. List two (2) AV blocks that may occur at the level of the bundle of His.
    1.
    2.

37. Identify the following rhythm:

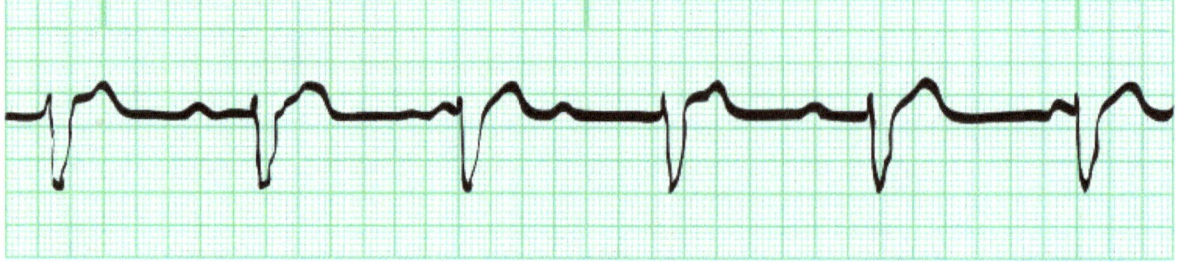

38. Identify the following rhythm:

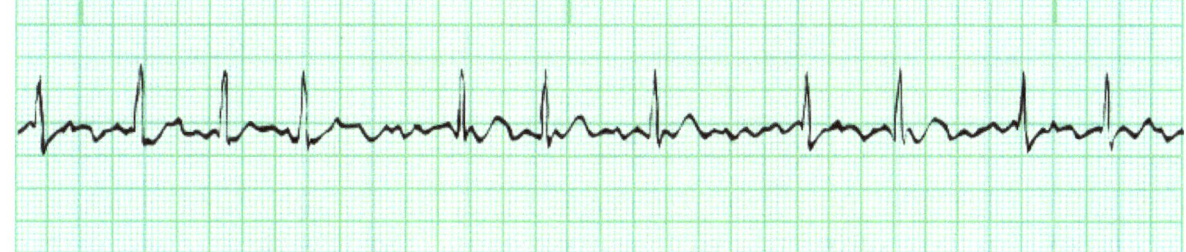

39. Identify the following rhythm:

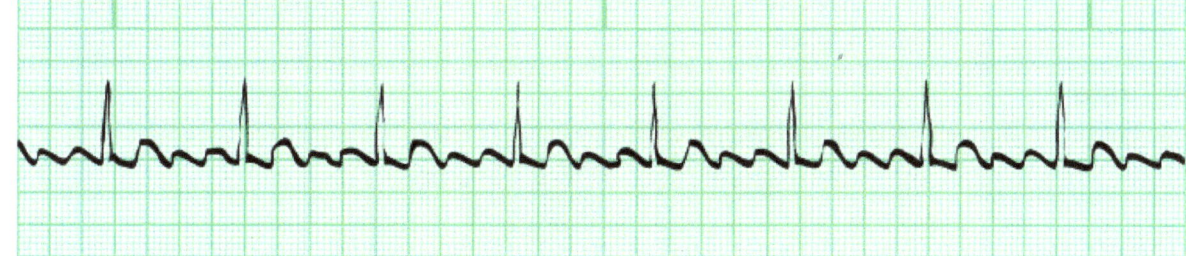

40. Identify the following rhythm:

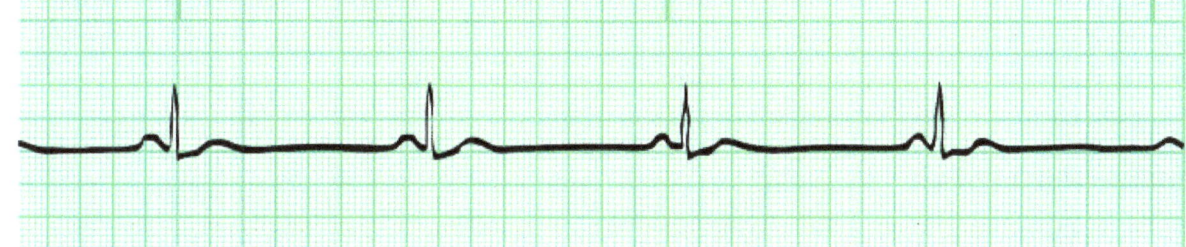

41. Identify the following rhythm:

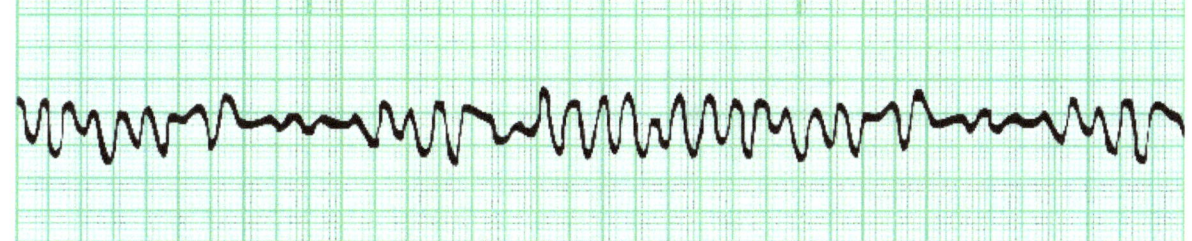

42. Identify the following rhythm:

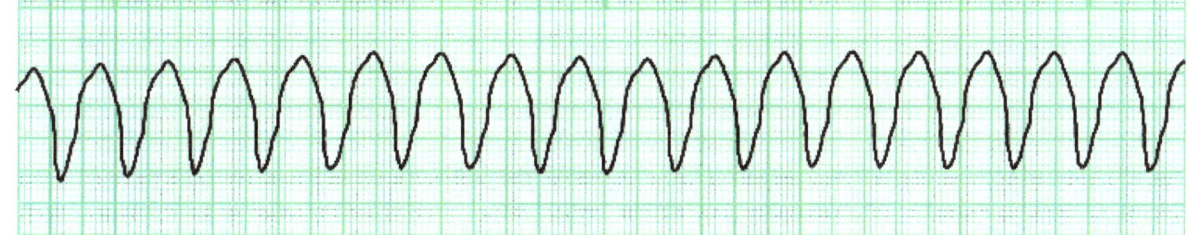

Common Cardiovascular Agents

One of the essentials of quality care of a patient who is having an acute myocardial infarction is pharmacological therapy. The following are the common pharmacological agents used.

Oxygen

Oxygen should be given to all patients with acute chest pain that may be due to cardiac ischemia, suspected hypoxemia of any cause, and cardiopulmonary arrest. Prompt treatment of the hypoxemia may prevent cardiac arrest. For patients breathing spontaneously, masks and nasal cannulas can be used to administer oxygen.

Epinephrine

Epinephrine is indicated in the management of cardiac arrest. The chance of successful defibrillation is enhanced by administration of epinephrine and proper oxygenation.

Isoproterenol (Isuprel)

Isoproterenol produces an overall increase in heart rate and myocardial contractility, but newer agents have replaced it in most clinical settings. It is contraindicated in the routine treatment of cardiac arrest.

Dopamine (Intropin)

Dopamine is indicated for significant hypotension in the absence of hypovolemia. Significant hypotension is present when systolic blood pressure is less than 90 mmHg with evidence of poor tissue perfusion, oliguria, or changes in mental status. It should be used at the lowest dose that produces adequate perfusion of vital organs.

Beta Blockers: Propranolol, Metoprolol, Atenolol, and Esmolol

Beta blockers reduce heart rate, blood pressure, myocardial contractility, and myocardial oxygen consumption which make them effective in the treatment of angina pectoris and hypertension. They are also useful in preventing atrial fibrillation, atrial flutter, and paroxysmal supra-ventricular tachycardia. Adverse effects of beta blockers are hypotension, congestive heart failure and broncho-spasm.

Lidocaine

Lidocaine is the drug of choice for the suppression of ventricular ectopy, including ventricular tachycardia and ventricular flutter. Excessive doses can produce neurological changes, myocardial depression, and circulatory depression. Neurological toxicity is manifested as drowsiness, disorientation, decreased hearing ability, paresthesia, and muscle twitching, and eventual seizures.

Verapamil

Verapamil is used in the treatment of paroxysmal supraventricular tachycardia (PSVT), effective in terminating more than 90% of episodes of PVST in adults and infants. Verapamil is also useful in slowing ventricular response to atrial flutter and fibrillation. Vigilant monitoring of blood pressure is recommended due to hypotension that could occur.

Digitalis

Digitalis increases the force of cardiac contraction as well as cardiac output.. Digitalis toxicity is common with an incidence of up to 20%. Patients require constant monitoring for signs and symptoms of toxicity such as: yellow vision, nausea, vomiting, and drowsiness.

Morphine Sulfate

It is the traditional drug of choice for the pain and anxiety associated with acute myocardial infarction. In high doses, morphine sulfate may cause respiratory depression. It is a controlled substance and has a tendency for abuse and addiction.

Nitroglycerin

Nitroglycerin is a powerful smooth muscle relaxant effective in relieving angina pectoris. It is effective for both exertional and rest angina. Headache is a common consequence following the administration of this drug. Hypotension may occur and patients should be instructed to sit or lie down while taking nitroglycerin.

Legal Considerations

Informed consent

This is consent given by the patient who is made aware of any procedure to be performed, its risks, expected outcomes, and alternatives.

Patient confidentiality

This is the key concept of HIPAA. All patients have a right to privacy and all information should remain privileged. Discuss patient information only with the patient's physician or office personnel that need certain information to do their job. Obtain a signed consent form to release medical information to the insurance company or other individual.

Negligence

This is the failure to exercise the standard of care that a reasonable person would give under similar circumstances and someone suffers injury because of another's failure to live up to a required duty of care.

    The four elements of negligence, (4 Ds), are:
1. Duty: duty of care
2. Derelict: breach of duty of care
3. Direct cause: legally recognizable injury occurs as a result of the breach of duty of care.
4. Damage: wrongful activity must have caused the injury or harm that occurred.

Tort
Is a wrongful act that results in injury to one person by another. Some examples of common torts that can occur in the clinic are the following:

- *Battery* - The basis of tort in this case is the unprivileged touching of one person by another. When a procedure is to be performed on a patient, the patient must give consent in full knowledge of the procedure and the risk it entails (informed consent).
- *Invasion of privacy* – This is the release of medical records without the patient's knowledge and permission.
- *Defamation of character* – This consists of injury to another person's reputation, name, or character through spoken (slander) or written (libel) words.

Good Samaritan Law - This law deals with the rendering of first aid by health care professionals at the scene of an accident or sudden injury. It encourages health care professionals to provide medical care within the scope of their training without fear of being sued for negligence.

Infection Control/Chain Of Infection
This consists of links, each of which is necessary for the infectious disease to spread. Infection control is based on the fact that the transmission of infectious diseases will be prevented or stopped when any level in the chain is broken or interrupted.

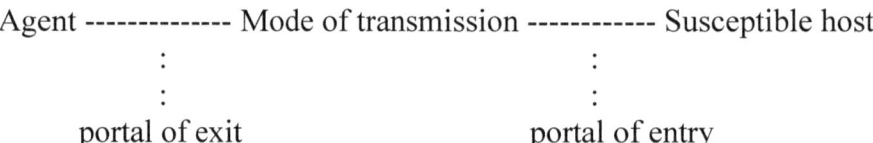

  Agent -------------- Mode of transmission ------------ Susceptible host
     :   :
     :   :
  portal of exit   portal of entry

 Agents – are infectious microorganisms that can be classified into groups namely: viruses, bacteria, fungi, and parasites. When infectious diseases are identified according to the specific disease-causing microorganism, the disease may be prevented with the use of anti-infective drugs or infection control practices.

 Portal of exit – the method by which an infectious agent leaves its reservoir. Standard Precautions and Transmission-Based Precautions are control measures aimed at preventing the spread of the disease as infectious agents exit the reservoir.

 Mode of transmission – specific ways in which microorganisms travel from the reservoir to the susceptible host. There are five main types of mode of transmission:
- Contact : direct and indirect
- Droplet
- Airborne
- Common vehicle
- Vectorborne

Portal of entry – allows the infectious agent access to the susceptible host. Common entry sites are broken skin, mucous membranes, and body systems exposed to the external environment such as the respiratory, gastrointestinal, and reproductive. Methods such as sterile wound care, transmission-based precautions, and aseptic technique limit the transmission of the infectious agents.

Susceptible host – The infectious agent enters a person who is not resistant or immune. Control at this level is directed towards the identification of the patients at risk, treat their underlying condition for susceptibility, or isolate them from the reservoir.

Medical Asepsis
Best defined as "the destruction of pathogenic microorganisms after they leave the body." It also involves environmental hygiene measures such as equipment cleaning and disinfection procedures. Methods of medical asepsis are Standard Precautions and Transmission-Based Precautions.

Handwashing
Hand washing is the most important means of preventing the spread of infection. A routine hand wash procedure uses plain soap to remove soil and transient bacterial. Hand antisepsis requires the use of antimicrobial soap to remove, kill or inhibit transient microorganisms. It is important that all healthcare personnel learn proper hand washing procedures.

Barrier Protection
Protective clothing provides a barrier against infection. Used properly, it will provide protection to the person wearing it; disposed of properly it will assist in the spread of infection. Learning how to put on and remove protective clothing is vital to insure the health and wellness of the person wearing the PPE. PPE's or personal protective equipment include:
- Masks
- Goggles
- Face Shields
- Respirator.

Isolation Precautions

For many years, the CDC recommended universal precautions, which is a method of infection control that assumed that all human blood and blody fluids were potentially infectious. The CDC issued a revised guidelines consisting of two tiers or levels of precautions: Standard Precautions and Transmission-Based Precautions.

Standard Precautions
This is an infection control method designed to prevent direct contact with blood and other body fluids and tissues by using barrier protection and work control practices. Under the standard precautions, all patients are presumed to be infective for blood-borne pathogens. Infection control practices to be used with all patients. These replace universal precautions and body substance isolation. They are used when there is a possibility of contact with any of the following:

- ◊ Blood
- ◊ All body fluids, secretions, and excretions (except sweat), regardless of whether or not they contain visible blood
- ◊ Nonintact skin
- ◊ Mucous membranes designed to reduce the risk of transmission of microorganisms from both
- ◊ Recognized and unrecognized sources of infections.

The standard precautions are:
- Wear gloves when collecting and handling blood, body fluids, or tissue specimen.
- Wear face shields when there is a danger for splashing on mucous membranes.
- Dispose of all needles and sharp objects in puncture-proof containers without recapping.

Transmission- Based Precautions the second tier of precautions and are to be used when the patient is known or suspected of being infected with contagious disease. They are to be used in addition to standard precautions. All types of isolation are condensed into three categories:

Contact precautions: are designed to reduce the risk of transmission of microorganisms by direct or indirect contact. Direct-contact transmission involves skin-to-skin contact and physical transfer of microorganisms to a susceptible host from an infected or colonized person. Indirect-contact transmission involves contact with a contaminated intermediate object in the patient's environment

Airborne precautions: are designed to reduce the risk of airborne transmission of infectious agents. Microorganisms carried in this manner can be dispersed widely by air currents and may become inhaled by or deposited on a susceptible host within the same room or over a longer distance from the source patient. Special air handling and ventilation are required to prevent airborne transmission.

Droplet precautions: are designed to reduce the risk of droplet transmission of infectious agents. Droplet transmission involves contact with the conjunctivae or the mucous membranes of the nose or mouth of a susceptible person with large-particle droplets generated from the source person primarily during coughing, sneezing, or talking. Because droplets generally travel only short distances, usually three feet or less, and do not remain suspended in the air, special air handling and ventilation are not required.

Latex Sensitivity

Latex sensitivity is an emerging and important problem in the health care field. Following the development of Universal Precaution Standards (OSHA, 1980), the use of natural rubber latex gloves for infection control skyrocketed. Within the last decade, however, the incidence of latex sensitivity has grown. Every health care worker must be concerned about latex sensitivity. Individuals with a known sensitivity to latex should wear a medical alert bracelet.

Legal Considerations

Informed consent: This is consent given by the patient who is made aware of any procedure to be performed, its risks, expected outcomes, and alternatives.

Patient confidentiality: This is the key concept of HIPAA. All patients have a right to privacy and all information should remain privileged. Discuss patient information only with the patient's physician or office personnel that need certain information to do their job. Obtain a signed consent form to release medical information to the insurance company or other individual.

Negligence: This is the failure to exercise the standard of care that a reasonable person would give under similar circumstances and someone suffers injury because of another's failure to live up to a required duty of care.
The four elements of negligence, (4 Ds), are:
1. Duty: duty of care
2. Derelict: breach of duty of care
3. Direct cause: legally recognizable injury occurs as a result of the breach of duty of care.
4. Damage: wrongful activity must have caused the injury or harm that occurred.

Tort: Is a wrongful act that results in injury to one person by another. Some examples of common torts that can occur in the clinic are the following:

Battery - The basis of tort in this case is the unprivileged touching of one person by another. When a procedure is to be performed on a patient, the patient must give consent in full knowledge of the procedure and the risk it entails (informed consent).

Invasion of privacy – This is the release of medical records without the patient's knowledge and permission.

Defamation of character – This consists of injury to another person's reputation, name, or character through spoken (slander) or written (libel) words.

Good Samaritan Law - This law deals with the rendering of first aid by health care professionals at the scene of an accident or sudden injury. It encourages health care professionals to provide medical care within the scope of their training without fear of being sued for negligence.

Resources:

Web Sites:
1. http://rnbob.tripod.com
2. http://davidge2.umaryland.edu
3. http://info.med.yale.edu
4. http://www.waycross.edu
5. http://www.usfca.edu

Reference books:
1. Principles of Clinical Electrocardiography, 13th edition, Goldschlager, Nora, MD.; Goldman Mervin J., MD
2. Basic Arrhythmias, 5th edition. Walraven, Gale
3. The only EKG Book You'll Ever Need, 4th Edition. Thaler, Malcom S., MD
4. Understanding 12-lead EKG's. Beasley, Brenda M., West, Michael C.,
5. ECG's Made Easy, 2nd Edition. Aehlert, Barbara
6. Gray's Anatomy. Gray, Henry. FRS., Carter, HV., MD

Sample EKG Exam

Choose the best answer:

1. A 60-year-old male patient has a history of on and off chest pain. His resting ECG is normal. It is decided to put him thru an exercise stress test. Which of the following will be the target heart rate for this patient?
    A. 180 beats per minute
    B. 160 beats per minute
    C. 140 beats per minute
    D. 120 beats per minute

2. This part of the conduction system of the heart is located at the superior portion of the interventricular septum and has the ability to function as a pacemaker with an intrinsic firing rate of 40-60 beats per minute.
    A. SA node
    B. AV node
    C. Bundle of His
    D. Purkinje fibers

3. This represents time it takes for electrical impulse to travel from the atria to the AV node, bundle of His, bundle branches and to the Purkinje fibers.
    A. PR interval
    B. PP interval
    C. RR interval
    D. QT interval

4. Which of the following is an indication for stress testing?
    A. Angina at rest
    B. Acute myocardial infarction
    C. Severe hypertension
    D. Evaluation of chest pain in a patient with normal baseline EKG

5. Which of the following is considered a negative Holter?
    A. Pauses
    B. Bradycardias or tachycardias
    C. No significant arrhythmias or ST changes.
    D. ST segment elevation or depression

6. The number of R waves in a six-second strip is 9. The heart rate is
    A. 72 per minute
    B. 45 per minute
    C. 90 per minute
    D. 54 per minute

7. Mr. Adam Edwards came to the clinic complaining of occasional chest pains, substernal in location and radiating to the left arm. The physician prescribed him medication to be taken during such chest pain episodes. A few days later, the patient came back with complain of headaches occurring after taking the medication. The medication prescribed is most likely:
   A. Procainamide
   B. Propranolol
   C. Nitroglycerin
   D. Digitalis

8. The following valves are called semilunar because they have half-moon shaped cusps:
   A. Pulmonic and tricuspid valves
   B. Aortic and mitral valves
   C. Pulmonic and mitral valves
   D. Aortic and pulmonic valves

9. Which of the following is incorrect of the augmented unipolar extremity leads?
   A. They represent the difference in the electrical potential between two extremities.
   B. The midpoint between two limbs is used as a negative reference point.
   C. Only one electrode from one limb makes a lead.
   D. The amplitude of deflections is increased by 50%.

10. This is an arrhythmia produced by an electrical impulse originating from a site other than the sinus node:
    A. Preexcitation syndromes
    B. Arrhythmia of sinus origin
    C. Conduction blocks
    D. Ectopic rhythms

11. Which of the following statements is incorrect regarding the limb leads?
    A. Electrodes and leads are applied to the right and left arms and legs.
    B. The right leg functions as a ground.
    C. The right leg plays a significant role in the production of the electrocardiogram.
    D. Where the electrode is placed in the extremities will make no difference in the electrical potential recorded.

12. The vertical axis of the EKG paper measures:
    A. Time
    B. Voltage/Amplitude
    C. Rhythm
    D. Heart rate

13. A normal PR interval should measure:
    A. .08 - .12 seconds
    B. < .12 seconds
    C. .12 - .20 seconds
    D. > .20 seconds

14. This electrode is place on the 4th intercostals space, left sternal border to create:
    A. V1
    B. V2
    C. V4
    D. V5

15. In a properly standardized EKG machine, 1mV should produce a deflection of:
    A. 10cm
    B. 10mm
    C. 1mm
    D. 0.1cm

16. Which of the following correctly describes P wave?
    A. This is thought to be due to repolarization of the Purkinje conduction system
    B. It is the deflection produced by atrial depolarization
    C. It is the deflection produced by ventricular depolarization
    D. It is the deflection produced by ventricular repolarization.

The sets of questions below consist of numbered items preceded by several lettered choices. For each numbered item select the **one** lettered choice with which it is **most** closely associated. Each lettered choice maybe used once, more than once, or not all.

A. SA Node	B. Internodal pathways
C. AV node	D. Bundle of His
E. Bundle branches	

17. _____ Located at the interventricular septum and conducts electrical impulse to the purkinje fibers
18. _____ There is a delay in electrical activity at this level allowing blood to flow from the atria to the ventricles

A. Lead I	B. Lead II
C. Lead III	D. aVR
E. aVL	

19. _____ The left arm is positive and the other limbs are negative
20. _____ The left arm is positive and the right arm is negative

Answer Key:

1. B	2. C	3. D	4. D	5. C
6. C	7. C	8. D	9. A	10. D
11. C	12. B	13. C	14. B	15. B
16. B	17. E	18. C	19. E	20. A

www.ingramcontent.com/pod-product-compliance
Lightning Source LLC
Chambersburg PA
CBHW050409180526

45159CB00005B/2205